Cancer & Heroes

By D Zeidler
© 2022

Executive summary:

The Bible dallies not, straightway encounter humanity's nature and the fray's front. But alas, Cain's failure becomes mythical in scope, broadcasting the forthcoming history of mankind. Was his battle against jealousy, envy, disparity, laziness, or pick your vice as it is not confided. Nor need it be, for the standard was efficiently revealed just four people into history.

> Genesis 4:6-7 The LORD said to Cain, "Why are you angry, and why has your face fallen? If you do well, will you not be accepted? And if you do not do well, sin is crouching at the door. Its desire is contrary to you, but you must rule over it."

The battle against our own interest and desires marches forth, though the terrain changes they align in our active will daily. The first salvo is seemingly innocuous as it is laid out in an unembellished inquiry, "Why?". "Why does God not want you to be like Him?"[1] Questioning, looking, understanding has allowed mankind to indeed be fruitful and multiply; "why" has been an asset.   The cost of inquiry is rarely tallied. Folly is at its utmost when the unexplainable or unknown is ceded as determinative. Trusting in

---

[1] Genesis 3:5 "For God knows that when you eat of it your eyes will be opened, and you will be like God, knowing good and evil."

the completeness of reason, God is terminated as "why" is left open.

God specifically addresses only two people in regards to their question of why, Job and Paul.[2] You can garner much by what people do not examine or consider. Any marginal Christian and still much of society is familiar with Job's circumstances and Paul's thorn. Most people find neither answer given by God satisfying. This is obvious today as God's response is disregarded, ignored, relegated aside as if it were an empty container. Any so-called attempt to seek answers to the human condition dearth of Job and Paul exposes the absolute primacy of man's experience. Unwilling to hear, many still seek answers to the unanswerable.

> Job 40:7 "Dress for action like a man; I will question you, and you make it known to me."

"Why" provides few spiritual solutions but whittles many unnecessary holes.   The pocketed field leftover from the unresolvable oft exposes the battlefield for decades and even lifetimes.

Opportunities in living are the hallmark of life. Some maybe pleasant, some unpleasant while the vast majority remain neutral. It is in the

---

[2] Moses will be presented and discussed. His situation is slightly different as he is not wanting relief or understanding of the situation. He is attempting to offer an excuse for not performing as God directs. He indirectly asks, "Why do you want me to lead when I am not well spoken?" He did not inquire, "Why am I made this way."

most unpleasant occurrences that the challenge
is brought to the forefront and the true mark of
courage is formed. Bravery can be found in your
actions addressing circumstances.

I believe it is harmful calling it a fight against
cancer or to bravely stand against a disability.
Most people are probably well meaning with
their praise and ignorant of consequences.
Hesitant to cast aspersions but we do arrogantly
both grant and convey a flattery in unearned
labels. Could it be just a desire to comfort
ourselves as those with imperfections are
elevated even though "the flawed" are just trying
to live. Be it well reasoned or not, as a
consequence, the true titles are diminished to
encourage the weak. And even if preemptively,
assumptively assigned these false labels only
reassure those in their grounding for asking
"why". There is no honor had in circumstances.
It is in actions and reactions whereby glory is
had. Honor is found in ruling over your desires.
Promulgating the meager wanting of life as an
extraordinary accomplishment belittles the act of
obedience to anything beyond ourselves. We
turn the battle lines around falsely finding an
enemy and pretending the normal is difficult.
Possessing a desire to live is ordinary.

Do you think about making your heart beat?
Can you? Living is easy, doing as we desire is
normal. Going against my wants forms the true
boundaries of the arena. Cancer may make it
harder to live but taking steps to continue life is
integral to the everyday regardless of

circumstances. Cancer is not a foreign invader; it is part of my body out of control. And but for outside intervention there is no possibility of control. Individuals born with bodily deformities, either internal or external, face the same situation: this was out of my control. Once you accept circumstances as a hinderance to living, the choices are the same for everyone. The desire to live is indeed a simple choice. Because you read, I can confidently say you have chosen to live.

Elevating the mundane is a common tack as old as history. Genesis 3:1 "Did God actually say, 'You shall not eat of any tree in the garden'?" Everything was available save for two trees. One rule, mundane, simple, and plain; yet, it was raised into the utmost of importance. "Did God say?", belittling the important is a standard opening when negation is the goal. Raising the common into a self-stylized epic occurrence lowers the ability to see the true battle. There is no battle against cancer, one does not bravely fight against cancer, I was not courageous undergoing chemotherapy. I, like you, just live.

Preface

I have a terminal cancer. One of the first
lessons to learn is how unique you are. Most
find this positively noteworthy but not so within
medicine. Not as criticism but as reality,
chances of success are merely guesses of what
might be. How my body responds to a treatment
is different than another person's physical
results and even how I might react a month from
now maybe different than today.

This acceptance of individuality makes forward
motion more readily available. Just as while
living without, so must my direction be with.
Rather than viewed as a death sentence, cancer
is just an opportunity for increases. As the
ancient Greeks formulated, in pain there can be
gain.

How do you define words? Most speak as they
hear. Your affiliations most likely form your
vernacular and its meanings. The importance of
defining often loses as priorities are rather
placed on communication within and acceptance
by a group.

Contained in these next few words the Bible's
definitions are given priority and the
consequences of this choice are discussed.

Table of Contents

Introduction:

> 1 Corinthians 15:55 "O death, where is your victory? O death, where is your sting?"

Where is the sting in death? What is the sting associated with dying? Is it a great unknown which haunts?[3] Is it the raw enjoyment of the earthly experience which we do not want to end? Or, are we fearful of what we have earned while living? Regardless, an examination of when man was first confronted, he chose knowledge over life.[4] Seemingly, it was in this newly gained knowledge which contained such a revelation as death became a horror. In the very beginning, though not known, information consisted of only the good. Recall the environment and the tempter's proposition of Adam and Eve, if death was a "sting" given from the moment of creation a choice between tree A.) good and evil, or tree B.) life; the decision would not have been difficult. Adam and Eve would have been tempted by life not by opened eyes.[5] It was within the knowledge of good and evil that death

---

[3] For the Christian there is great comfort as it is not unknown. Luke 23:43 "And he said to him, "Truly, I say to you, today you will be with me in paradise."

[4] Genesis 3:22 "Then the LORD God said, "Behold, the man has become like one of us in knowing good and evil. Now, lest he reach out his hand and take also of the tree of life and eat, and live forever—"

[5] Genesis 3:5 "For God knows that when you eat of it your eyes will be opened, and you will be like God, knowing good and evil."

gained its sting. Had obedience been, death would not. Knowledge brought forth consequences that, though revealed, they refused to grasp. The introduction of imperfection in a realm of perfections immediately brought shame.[6] And birthed from shame the Lord God was avoided. The lawless attempt to escape judgement. And death had victory in the first battle.

The Christian proclamation of victory over death rightly evokes a conquering. For salvation we must conquer over the knowledge gained by Adam and Eve; that is, we must decide to freely live in obedience. The freedom of choice is so alluring that even today mankind still chooses death over life.[7] But unlike Adam and Eve the horror is apparent for those alive today, for in their exposing of knowledge death's sting was shown. Eternal punishment or heavenly comfort with the Maker.

Cancer, terrible illness, other defects are all seen as removing choice. Dying at an old age is the desired; as it is the preservation of choice for as long as possible. It is that choice which man

---

[6] Genesis 3:7-8 "Then the eyes of both were opened, and they knew that they were naked. And they sewed fig leaves together and made themselves loincloths. [8] And they heard the sound of the LORD God walking in the garden in the cool of the day, and the man and his wife hid themselves from the presence of the LORD God among the trees of the garden."

[7] Romans 1:20 "For his invisible attributes, namely, his eternal power and divine nature, have been clearly perceived, ever since the creation of the world, in the things that have been made. So, they are without excuse."

treasures above all else. Yet, freedom is removed when breath is no more. Regardless of age the sting of certain judgement reigns. While the Christian knowledge of salvation dampens the reality, it stings despite. Do not be deceived as Christ willingly showed the effects of the sting.[8]

Have empathy for those tasting the sting, staring at the abyss, those who have tried but cannot avoid claiming an excuse that never was; pity these for it is in this knowledge, death is feared. Weep with the helpless as the past cannot change for their ancient awareness is "clearly" embedded. Comfort those whose shame now knows no relief. Pray that in their pain the house of mirth is empty.[9] The word of the truth is that which can set men free from the sting.[10]

Within their knowledge mankind adapted the language of war, death is to be avoided and so a battle was created. The wrong foe is feared; the end is dreaded while the tempter is enjoyed. Fight bravely and courageously against the inevitable is the odd adopted mantra. Rather, we should battle against desires as sin crouches in wait. As heirs of the legacy descended from Adam and Eve, we too know the shame, still

---

[8] John 11:35 "Jesus wept."

[9] Ecclesiastes 7:4 "The heart of the wise is in the house of mourning, but the heart of fools is in the house of mirth."

[10] John 8:31-32 "So Jesus said to the Jews who had believed him, "If you abide in my word, you are truly my disciples, and you will know the truth, and the truth will set you free.""

today humanity seeks the avoidance of the Lord God's judgment.

Part I

Detours occur throughout your life, does a detour define you or merely offer some limitation? During a vacation trip as we traveled far off the network of the interstate complex and even away from the highway system, we encountered a detour. Emergency water line repairs were underway resulting in the road having a temporary ditch. This ditch forced a 20-minute roundabout path to be taken. Suppose instead, we were the first ones to discover the water line rupture and did so by plunging into the newly eroded crevice. The wrecked vehicle would be no longer able to travel. Then the vacation plans would have needed to be altered more than a 20-minute drive around. Or suppose we arrived at this location 1 hour later and the road way had been repaired, we would have never known. A broken water line brought forth an unexpected limitation and the necessary adjustments. Timing could have made this event significantly different. Why did this happen to us? Is God punishing someone in this vehicle? Our reaction was neither brave nor courageous rather we merely responded. And this is living encapsulated. Rarely do we ask, "Why did this rather mundane event occur?". Why should we? Things happen and we adjust.

Occasionally, the circumstances of the limitations can appear overwhelming and insurmountable. It is in these situations that many slip into aggrandized prideful self-centeredness, attributes become claimed either by self-assertions or bestowment. Attempts to answer the unanswerable bring frustration and confusion. Why did this happen to me? And in spite, many people giddily assign the random as deserved. Most are willing to accept that the rain falls on the just and the unjust[11]... until it happens to me and then there must be a reason.

I refuse to be defined by the uncontrollable, my mistakes, or even by others. I choose to live and because I am living things happen, mistakes are made and snapshots taken. The sun rises and the rain falls, be I just or unjust. However, these happenings should be seen merely as happenings. But in our narcissism, we hold ourselves apart. Superlatives are part of the everyday vernacular; dumbest, worst, best, strangest, and weirdest begins to form the impression. It is indeed common to turn everyday into the extraordinary. Hubris is easily found as it seems to dwell comfortably near the tongue of most.

The ancients described a good story in such terms; catharsis, a cleansing or purging by seeing like or better people succumb to everyday circumstances exaggerated by their own decisions. It is believed that this formula for catharsis is popular because a viewer can easily state, "I'm not that bad" or "I would never...". And when circumstances are devoid of decision

---

[11] Matthew 5:45 "... For he makes his sun rise on the evil and on the good, and sends rain on the just and on the unjust."

points it seems many people find elevation, promoting others as a misguided way to express gratitude this isn't happening to them. However, would I be considered "brave" because a tree branch fell on my toe and I was determined to walk again? Should I be considered "fighting" as I learn how to sing proficiently? Is it courageous because I just want to make the most out of today? At what point is living considered merely normal compared to something exemplary? Moving forward with your life should not be thought of as anything but ordinary.

Who decided to make bravery, fighting, and courageous associated with cancer? This question has several layers. The unknowable, trying to assign a who or maybe a time period. It also has a sentiment of why should I care. It is also expressed in a manner which most people would not give a second thought about; it is rigged up in importance and meaning because of everyone's close association with excessive self-pride, hubris. The underlying arrogance is a belief that one person can decide. Yes, one person had to have first used this phrase but it is only because of others; its ability to resonate throughout other individuals, did it take on a significance.   The "who" of who first said it, is not important. There are many such questions which really are not important in fact hurt or hinder thought. A better approach: I wonder why people are willing to or why do they use terms of confrontation when talking about more strenuous circumstances?

Part IB

Contrary to the mindset of most, the mere asking of a question does not create an obligation. There may not be a definitive why. Shifting the focus slightly, too many believe that God is comparable to a wish granting vending machine;[12] by putting in the correct sum in, a fulfillment comes out. Asking God for an answer and God will provide. Questions from you do not create obligations upon others. The most famously adopted version of this falsehood originates in the Bible: Matthew 7:7 "Ask, and it will be given to you; seek, and you will find; knock, and it will be opened to you." Of course, the solution, the caveat, is found just two verses later. Matthew 7:9 "Or which one of you, if his son asks him for bread, will give him a stone?" What parent is going to give their child something harmful? The Bible tells that God can and will answer a request but He need not. There is not a contract made merely because of a request or a question. The Bible directly states God will not provide harmful material. And who amongst us can say what is harmful and what is not? Who gives their child a snake when a loaf of bread is needed?   And do you know if you need a snake or a loaf?   Regardless, a question does not necessitate an answer. In practice asking "why" often causes bitterness to develop.

---

[12] Matthew 21:22 "And whatever you ask in prayer, you will receive, if you have faith."

To linger a bit on the idea of ask and you shall receive, consider King David and his prayer for healing.[13] 2 Samuel 12:16 "David therefore sought God on behalf of the child. And David fasted and went in and lay all night on the ground." David sought and received forgiveness for his sin. David pleaded with God to the point others were concerned about David's wellbeing. Yet, God did not relent. The child died. 2 Samuel 12:22-23 "He said, 'While the child was still alive, I fasted and wept, for I said, 'Who knows whether the LORD will be gracious to me, that the child may live?' But now he is dead. Why should I fast? Can I bring him back again? I shall go to him, but he will not return to me.'" First, through David's suffering we learn of a great assurance regarding heaven and the death of an infant. Second, David's prayer was not answered; asking did not make an obligation. Third, David knew he was appealing to the graciousness of God. Aren't we all appealing for the gracious mercy of God in any request we make upon the Almighty? Fourth, the child lingered in life for seven days. Too many would declare God cruel for allowing this poor child to suffer that long. Why would God do such a mean thing? "Why" is a dangerous question to pose to God. Fifth, after his child's death David did not linger in the past, he simply moved forward. To be clear, God told David of this punishment. We are not given such insights. Still, the Bible is consistent from Genesis to

---

[13] 2 Samuel 12:14 "Nevertheless, because by this deed you have utterly scorned the LORD, the child who is born to you shall die."

Revelation. The famous ask and it shall be is not an open-ended promise.

To further expand, consider the book of Hebrews and the eleventh chapter verses 37 to 40:

> "They were stoned, they were sawn in two, they were killed with the sword. They went about in skins of sheep and goats, destitute, afflicted, mistreated— of whom the world was not worthy—wandering about in deserts and mountains, and in dens and caves of the earth. And all these, though commended through their faith, did not receive what was promised, since God had provided something better for us, that apart from us they should not be made perfect."

They did not receive as prayed for. God does, can, and will answer prayer. However, God's timing, ways and methods do not need to correspond with our considerations. The bounds of your ego find no edge if God's answers are believed foreseeable.

Recall Paul and his thorn. He asked, he requested, and he solicited again without resolution. Still, some want to claim it is because of human error that God does not respond. Are you willing to cast aspersions on Paul in order to force God into a box? Such self-import is utter folly. God will have mercy as He desires. [14] Paul's desire was indeed strong but

God would not respond according to Paul's longing. Praying to God, communicating with the Maker should not be taken lightly. God hears, listens, and responds to His creation. Like many human foibles we push beyond the limits into the realm of declaring power over God, reducing Him to a small "g".

> 2 Corinthians 12:7-10 So to keep me from becoming conceited because of the surpassing greatness of the revelations, a thorn was given me in the flesh, a messenger of Satan to harass me, to keep me from becoming conceited. Three times I pleaded with the Lord about this, that it should leave me. But he said to me, "My grace is sufficient for you, for my power is made perfect in weakness." Therefore I will boast all the more gladly of my weaknesses, so that the power of Christ may rest upon me. For the sake of Christ, then, I am content with weaknesses, insults, hardships, persecutions, and calamities. For when I am weak, then I am strong.

Do not be conceited enough to think God will give as you ask or answer as you desire. Paul was fortunate in that he knew the why...but, it still changed not his desire. Do you think knowing "why" would really help you cope with what has befallen you? Paul still wanted this thorn removed. "Why" does not provide relief.

---

[14] Romans 9:18 "So then he has mercy on whomever he wills, and he hardens whomever he wills."

Posing questions to God is a "clever" way of
rebelling. Unanswerable questions are just ways
to hide self-centeredness. Just as with Paul,
even if you knew "why" it would not change your
desire. Three times Paul asked. Three times
God said no. Do not think yourself in greater
harmony with God's desires than Paul. You of
strong ego take note, ask and you shall receive
is not a magic genie responding to your beckon
free of consequences and unable to see beyond
meager earthly insights.

Part II

I am not fighting cancer; perhaps, one could say
that I fight to live to the fullest. Struggle, not to
live longer but to live. I "fought" to live before I
became ill and though the path is now different
the methods remain. Do not attempt to relegate
compassion, empathy or sympathy into cliches
of supposed elevation. Nobleness is not found
by wanting to live; rather, life is only possibly
noble in what you live for. Associative projection
of accomplishment for the normative reaction or
action is insulting. The weak of intellect
embrace elevation regardless of the factual. In
reality it is belittling to intitle the undeserved.

History books do not note normal, everyday
behavior. We know very little concerning daily
life of an ordinary African, Asian, Englishman,
or a European 700 years ago. It is the
aberration which is recorded. The "heroes" or
the "villains" from the past find their way into
the annals. Those that did not fit into the mold
of the common are considered courageous or
brave. We want to be recorded; we want to be
noted. Of course, we will use self-inflating
superlatives when allowed.

Bravery and courage describe actions that
should be but are not regularly observed. Is an
animal brave for wanting to live? Is a worm
courageous for wiggling off a drying concrete
pad? The normative is to adjust in order to live.
The ordinary is to be alive. It is odd not to strive

for living despite circumstances. Therefore, by a truer context and usage heroes do what non-heroes won't. The worm is not heroic as it struggles as any other worm would likewise do. Mankind is not brave because he just wants to live. History will not title or label me courageous for "fighting" against cancer.

The Bible gives an appropriately differing definition to nobility, courage and bravery than the one thus far described as prescribed while being ill or born with impediments to being "normal". Matthew 16:24-25 "Then Jesus told his disciples, 'If anyone would come after me, let him deny himself and take up his cross and follow me. For whoever would save his life will lose it, but whoever loses his life for my sake will find it.'" It is the average to pursue self-preservation it is the abnormal not to follow this course. Humanity desires its own ways and wishes. And in this present context living is very much a part of the human's desired path. Unless we prefer for everyone to be worthily titled "brave", it is in the following of God's commands that the noble is revealed. It is the denial of self which is brave. Christ tells how people try to save their own life; this is the normal course of human action. Christ also told His followers to deny themselves; again, because this is not normal behavior. Accordingly, it is in denial that you are actually fighting. And true rebuffing of self is brave.

"He bravely fought cancer for several years..." or "Throughout her life she courageously battled against the limitations imposed at her birth." To be consistent with current usage the same sentiments can be said of a mouse. Did the mouse battle through being born with 3 legs? Did the mouse bravely struggle to escape from the trap? Titles and words by necessity have meaning, language and even society demands that yes, means yes.[15] We diminish the important in order to feed the ego. Surviving is not brave. Similarly, the ordinary desire to survive is not courageous. It is, however, courageous to fight against your own self-interest; heroism is not found in the pursuit of self-preservation. According to the words found in Matthew it is normal to pursue that which you desire and only different to deny yourself. Using a bombastic militaristic rhetoric illustrates how little we deny ourselves; self-aggrandizement only elevates the ego. Perhaps some find comfort in self-deception, maybe some convince themselves in the foolery of wordsmithing that they are now greater than, but I find not.

Regarding the interpersonal, the Bible speaks in a tone which contradicts the vernacular developed in a hospital ward. Everyone experiences a battle as Biblically defined. It speaks of a grim challenging personal effort against the unknown. Ephesians 6:12 "For we do not wrestle against flesh and blood, but against the rulers, against the authorities,

---

[15] James 5:12 "But above all, my brothers, do not swear, either by heaven or by earth or by any other oath, but let your "yes" be yes and your "no" be no, so that you may not fall under condemnation."

against the cosmic powers over this present darkness, against the spiritual forces of evil in the heavenly places." Do not be deceived or belittle Paul's description, the oldest book in the Bible begins offering a narrative to such a spiritual battle. Job 1:6-7 "Now there was a day when the sons of God came to present themselves before the LORD, and Satan also came among them. The LORD said to Satan, "From where have you come?" Satan answered the LORD and said, "From going to and fro on the earth, and from walking up and down on it."

The devil, and we believe his other cosmic followers, go to and fro and it is on this front from which we wage a battle, demonstrate courage, show bravery. We do not wrestle against a desire to live; we wrestle against a desire to become our own arbitrator. We fight the temptation of denying or challenging, "Is this what God really said?"[16] As recorded among the first words spoken was the desire of the self. I want. We want to decide right and wrong. It is distinctive to desire other than I. Be not led astray by a false descriptive language of triumph, there is no battle against cancer. I want to live; therefore, I pursue as I pursue.

The treatment of my particular cancer involves travails, pain and distress upon my body and mind. Currently, chemotherapies do kill the harmful cells but often reach beyond the target.

---

[16] Genesis 3:1 "Now the serpent was more crafty than any other beast of the field that the LORD God had made. He said to the woman, "Did God actually say, 'You shall not eat of any tree in the garden'?"

Killing is an accurate term just as one kills a
mouse but it happens not in a battle. Though
the term killing is precise, there is not active
consideration occurring, there are no
combatants. The medicine does as it was
designed. Medicine does not consider if its
actions are right or wrong, it reacts as a ball
falls to the ground when dropped. The cancer
does not plot a counter-offensive. A flame is not
battling a container of water, deciding how to
best distribute its heat neither is chemo trying to
figure out if this "attack" should be modified to
best achieve the desired results. The physicians
are not generals though they order much
movement of resources. Society is full of tools
which can accomplish various tasks and are
often narrow in scope. A stereotypical regular
hammer is efficient at transferring energy but
horrible at promoting vegetive growth.
Chemicals that destroy cancer are just like a
mindless hammer used by my body. Other than
consent I put forth no physical effort in order for
the treatment to effect. A doctor prescribes and
directs like a general but the orders do not have
participants that must likewise make decisions.
The medicine does not need a word of
encouragement in order to proceed.   A nurse
does not risk their life in order to deliver the
destructive medicine. Yes, chemo therapy kills
but what occurs inside my body does not qualify
as a battle. It is merely the results of a chemical
reaction to which my body responds.

Wanting to live is not courageous. Bravery is not found in inaction. A fight is not found amongst chemicals.

We do not live riskless rather we mitigate and manage potentialities. Contrary to a modern conception, every medical intervention has the prospective for the undesired. There are always risks and odds of failures and success. Is consideration of the rewards compared to the risk bravery or logic? Do probabilities demand courage to assess or are they just common sense? Specifically, prudent behaviors need not be universal. Unacceptable risk for one person maybe acceptable for another. And for two differing people who choose two differing paths neither maybe "wrong". One who decides on treatment does not earn the title of brave while the other who does not is not a coward.

Though not yet mentioned, the opposite of bravery is cowardness. You never hear, "The reason they died is because they were such a coward by not fighting cancer better." We are quick to assign the heroic and cancer together but nary present anyone as cowardly. To use a game analogy, losers must be for winners to be had. Winning has no meaning but for losing. Bravery, likewise, must have two identifiable oppositions. The normal behavior and the cowardly behavior for comparison. To illustrate simply: it is normal to stand, it is brave to run towards, and it is cowardly to run away. Another way to see the falsehood in titling someone as brave for their decisions regarding a birth defect, cancer, or another such aliment is the lack of reference of coward. Without a comparison some words are meaningless in practice.

You do not fight against a disability. You may struggle more than the average person to accomplish some tasks. But that is not properly fighting, it is living. The disability does not plan how to counter your adjustments it just is present. You are not brave for seeking a treatment to live longer despite the consequences. You are merely making a choice to try and live. Are you brave to go and buy food in order to live? Are you courageous in sleeping? The necessary to live should not be considered significant. Terms matter both temporally and eternally.

Language is far more fragile than might be apparent. While the truth endures much the danger in the assignment of elevated falsified titles to benign events belies its damage for belittling the truth. We fight against our personal desires and against disobedience to God. We wrestle against the evil spiritual forces in heavenly places. Reducing a challenge to God into semantics with a falsified "why" repeats the serpents, "Did God really say?" and ignores God's response of "Where were you?"[17] Do not belittle that battle. Perhaps this verse can take on greater significance: Job 38:2 "Who is this

---

[17] Job 38:4 "Where were you when I laid the foundation of the earth? Tell me, if you have understanding.

that darkens counsel by words without
knowledge?"

Part III

> Romans 8:28 "And we know that for those who love God all things work together for good, for those who are called according to his purpose."

And the foolish among us want to know why, find justification, find reasoning, believing that understanding matters? Would any justification be reasonable? Why did this happen? The "why" is a poor disguise for the inquiry: How am I important? Of the billions of people this befalling on me must be significant. Seeking meaning for existence is pure futility, void of the Devine. And in the Almighty's shadow we exist; oddly befuddled, just as Adam was unwilling to accept a simple rule, we are averse to accept a basic role and insist to proceed with the same question of "why God would…?" Sadly, history is replicated.

"Were you there?" is God's response to Job; He did not answer "all things work for good." It is far more reasonable to draw an inference from God's response to Job than it does to Christ's response to His disciples. Do you honestly think God is going to heal in such a fashion that two thousand years from now you will be referenced just as the blind man from long ago is?[18] Do you find it satisfying to know why God allowed

---

[18] John 9:3 "Jesus answered, "It was not that this man sinned, or his parents, but that the works of God might be displayed in him."

Satan to torment Job?[19] No, you do not. An
answer to the wrong question does not provide
relief.

And God's answers of "where were you" and "all
things for good" are not contradictory; rather,
they correctly change the emphasis or the
inquiry and answer two separate questions.

It is easy to understand that God's specific
command to Adam and Eve regarding two trees
is no longer applicable. It is easy to understand
that God's directive to build an ark[20] is not an
imperative to you. Unfortunately, we tussle
separating the specific from the universal;
extracting as we want.   And this is particularly
true when you seek reassurances and comfort
from Bible passages.

Romans 8:19 "For the creation waits with eager
longing for the revealing of the sons of God."
Yes, all things work for the eternal good for
believers; we, like the rest of creation, eagerly

---

[19] Job 1:8-11 "And the LORD said to Satan, "Have you considered my
servant Job, that there is none like him on the earth, a blameless and
upright man, who fears God and turns away from evil?" Then Satan
answered the LORD and said, "Does Job fear God for no reason? Have
you not put a hedge around him and his house and all that he has, on
every side? You have blessed the work of his hands, and his
possessions have increased in the land. But stretch out your hand and
touch all that he has, and he will curse you to your face."
[20] Genesis 6:13-14 "And God said to Noah, "I have determined to make
an end of all flesh, for the earth is filled with violence through them.
Behold, I will destroy them with the earth. [14] Make yourself an ark
of gopher wood. Make rooms in the ark, and cover it inside and out
with pitch."

waits for His second coming. This unique good
in verse 28 is not about your specific
circumstances being resolved presently in a
manner conducive to your understanding. The
Bible concludes a listing of the faithful with this
note of earthly misery. Hebrews 11:36 "Others
suffered mocking and flogging, and even chains
and imprisonment." All things do work for and
towards the fulfillment of prophesies and
awaiting the way for Christ's second coming.
Mankind detects little beyond the lids attached
above their visual orbs. The "good" in Romans
8:28 need not apply to your earthly knowledge.

All questions are not benign. Any attempt to
reconcile God's plan with the human condition
devoid of God's answer to Job should be
rejected. Why did this happen? By the asking
of "why", you are now the faultfinder.   The
Christian's answer is simple: Because it
happened. Job 40:2 "Shall a faultfinder contend
with the Almighty? He who argues with God, let
him answer it." Job 40:8 "Will you even put me
in the wrong? Will you condemn me that you
may be in the right?" We are not told why; we
are told what to do. Glorify God.[21] Jesus knew
why the man in John 9 was blind from birth;
God had prepared for that particular moment so

---

[21] Isaiah 45:8-9 "Shower, O heavens, from above, and let the clouds
rain down righteousness; let the earth open, that salvation and
righteousness may bear fruit; let the earth cause them both to sprout;
I the LORD have created it. "Woe to him who strives with him who
formed him, a pot among earthen pots! Does the clay say to him who
forms it, 'What are you making?' or 'Your work has no handles'?"

that Christ could choose to demonstrate God's works.

> John 9:2-4 "And his disciples asked him, "Rabbi, who sinned, this man or his parents, that he was born blind?" Jesus answered, "It was not that this man sinned, or his parents, but that the works of God might be displayed in him. We must work the works of him who sent me while it is day; night is coming, when no one can work."

From a human perspective, why was this man blind? Because he was. No one sinned, no one caused this event, it just happened. When Christ with Godly insight arrived the true purpose of this individuals' circumstances were revealed. The lesson for today from this event long ago is to learn not to ask "why" but rather ask how can this or how can I glorify Christ. Things happen which present opportunities for you to glorify God. It rains on the just and equally on the unjust.[22] There truly may not be a "why" rather it is an opportunity to glorify God with your praises.

Romans 8:18 "For I consider that the sufferings of this present time are not worth comparing with the glory that is to be revealed to us." According to Paul there is no comparison between our present suffering and the eternal

---

[22] Matthew 5:45 "so that you may be sons of your Father who is in heaven. For he makes his sun rise on the evil and on the good, and sends rain on the just and on the unjust."

glory of God. All things work for the good isn't
an answer for "why"; rather, it changes your
focus away from yourself to the eternal. Romans
8:28 isn't about you and your situation per se; it
is about your choice to whom to glorify. Romans
8:28 "And we know that for those who love God
all things work together for good, for those who
are called according to his purpose." Note, verse
29 confirms the eternal over the temporal;
Romans 8:29 "For those whom he foreknew he
also predestined to be conformed to the image of
his Son, in order that he might be the firstborn
among many brothers." Ignoring the topic of
"predestined" for this matter, it is clear that
"predestined to be conformed to the image of his
Son" is speaking of the eternal and not attaining
perfection here on earth. Yes, all things do work
together bringing conformity via eternal life.
This verse is not about the "why" of present
circumstances rather it is about eternal hope.

Paul repeats this same message to the
Corinthians, how these earthly suffering are not
comparable to eternal glory. 2 Corinthians 4:17
"For this light momentary affliction is preparing
for us an eternal weight of glory beyond all
comparison...". And this message is the same
throughout the Bible.

Do not claim your "suffering" is something larger
than an opportunity for you to glorify God, there
is nothing larger. Psalms 102:18 "Let this be
recorded for a generation to come, so that a
people yet to be created may praise the LORD".
The Psalmist makes this clear, the Bible is

recorded for generations to come, that is you. You have now been created. You are not naturally a continuation of the past. The Bible is recorded so that you may know of God's works, guidance and commands. And this record is presented so that you may praise the Lord. There is nothing new under the sun which will befall you, it all has been.[23] It is recorded for you to give your praise and honor where it is due.[24]

Whatever has/will befalls you is an opportunity for you to display God's power over your life.

The elevating of self by claiming to battle a life-threatening illness is foolish. Your desire to live is normal, we battle to praise God despite circumstances. It is easy to praise God when all is well. God acknowledge this truth to Satan. Job 1:12 "And the LORD said to Satan, "Behold, all that he has is in your hand. Only against him do not stretch out your hand." So Satan went out from the presence of the LORD." Accept what comes without a "why" but with a "what"; what can I do now?

Perhaps you can see this point most succinctly in James where this is stated. Your faith is

---

[23] Ecclesiastes 1:9 "What has been is what will be, and what has been done is what will be done, and there is nothing new under the sun."
[24] 1 Peter 1:6-7 "In this you rejoice, though now for a little while, if necessary, you have been grieved by various trials, so that the tested genuineness of your faith—more precious than gold that perishes though it is tested by fire—may be found to result in praise and glory and honor at the revelation of Jesus Christ."

tested. So, how will you respond to this testing.
Will you count it joy or become bitter? Will you
glorify your maker or wallow in the self-pity
surrounding the question beginning with "why"?

> James 1:2-3 "Count it all joy, my brothers,
> when you meet trials of various kinds, for
> you know that the testing of your faith
> produces steadfastness."

In John chapter 11, readers are told Jesus'
friend, Lazarus was dying of an illness. Lazarus'
family was gravely concerned and sent word to
Jesus of the situation. And then to expound on
several points germane to these presented within
chapter 11. Jesus waited two days before
leaving to go see Lazarus.[25] What would you
think if you were Mary or Martha waiting upon
Christ? God rarely works within our time frame.

> John 11:4 But when Jesus heard it he
> said, "This illness does not lead to death.
> It is for the glory of God, so that the Son of
> God may be glorified through it."

"This illness does not lead to death." Christ
knew the future and how He was going to
respond. Particularly notice the brief phrase,
"this illness", meaning another illness may kill
him. This was not a pronouncement of Lazarus
never dying in the future. "This illness" confines
components to that period. We should be clear
that some of Christ's actions and words in this

---

[25] John 11:6 "So, when he heard that Lazarus was ill, he stayed two
days longer in the place where he was."

circumstance apply only to this story. Intended with all respect and honor, it appears Jesus delayed going to Lazarus in order to maximize the effect of His healing. This particular healing would be done for two exacting goals. The first is that God the Father may be glorified. Given other scriptures and consideration of the events present in the story, the glorification of God is not confined to this healing or moment in history. We can glorify God in our circumstances. The second goal was to glorify the Son.

> John 11:45 "Many of the Jews therefore, who had come with Mary and had seen what he did, believed in him"

Jesus made disciples, followers, believers with His words, His claims, actions, and His promises. In John 11:15 we find these words, "I am glad I was not there, so that you may believe." Many of His actions were indeed for those moments in time so that His message would spread through those who believed. Jesus did not advocate for us to delay in rendering comfort and assistance where we can. The night has arrived, we cannot raise the dead.[26] Our actions tell of our beliefs. Christ did this miracle to glorify the Father and also Himself, the Son. We, in our capacity, have the same task.

---

[26] John 9:4 "We must work the works of him who sent me while it is day; night is coming, when no one can work."

Scripture is unified, pointing directly to our task: we are to glorify God. Jesus knew and explained the "why" regarding Lazarus. Does verse four mean that God caused his illness, "It is for the glory of God."? Or, does this mean that Christ knowing His future response will use this event to glorify.[27] For this purpose, it matters not. We cannot say if God directed your illness to occur. We cannot state that God caused you to be born with a disability.   I cannot state that God caused my illness to occur. It rains on the just and the unjust. Do not be deceived. Believe as you wish, your response and obligation changes not. Praise God. Glorify the Maker. To paraphrase verse four, "This happened, glorify the Father." You will not know the "why" but you do know your task. You do not know tomorrow but you do know eternity. The unknown often overrides the known. Resist this course.

"Fear God and keep His commandments."[28] Thus, Solomon summed the duty of man.

---

[27] While significantly larger than the scope intended here. It is not limiting to God that He can have the world function both "independently" and dependently. Raining on the just and unjust could be stating that God allows the world to function as he designed it, much like an automobile engine. Or the rain could be God's direct hand involved but applied evenly to believers and unbelievers alike. And there are myriads of other possibilities none of which necessarily change the belief in God's absolute sovereignty. The primary point intended here is the emphasis of glorifying God the Maker. Unlike Christ, we are greatly limited in knowledge. Do not become waylaid by "cause" which is just another term for the inquiry of "why". Our task remains the same with or without understanding of circumstances.

Irrespective of what befalls, humanity's task remains. "When this happens, then do as you please" is not an instruction given. An excuse for self-idolatry is swiftly embraced when an event differing from the normal besets. Solomon succinctly tied one common excuse, fear, into its corrected path. The fear of God should keep our path on obedience.

Very briefly, almost forced as the words of Solomon resonates, "fear" needs a slight explanation as it fits the overall discussion of the heroic. Frequently fear is used to manipulate, assigning importance to the normal with the intent to elevate circumstance, diminishing the truth. Fear should not be seen solely as a negative response to thoughts. The fear of God can motivate proper behavior. Fearing of the incorrect can lead away from commandments.

Fear is regularly viewed as a negative personal attribute; it does not, however, suffer ridicule from society. Some are regular practitioners of fear as they are even applauded though facts are shoved about like flakes in the wind. Fear of the incorrect is frequently cherished. I can imagine many unknowns. Let not the unknown guide you. Fear, if viewed as a title, fits well into this present writing; if miss applied, fear diminishes away from its intended purpose co-opted instead to elevate the enemy. Fear of tomorrow does not allow today to be compromised.

---

[28] Ecclesiastes 12:13 "The end of the matter; all has been heard. Fear God and keep his commandments, for this is the whole duty of man."

Revelation 14:7 "And he said with a loud voice, "Fear God and give him glory, because the hour of his judgment has come, and worship him who made heaven and earth, the sea and the springs of water."

Revelation 2:10 "Do not fear what you are about to suffer. Behold, the devil is about to throw some of you into prison, that you may be tested, and for ten days you will have tribulation. Be faithful unto death, and I will give you the crown of life."

Part IV

> Exodus 4:10-11 "But Moses said to the LORD, "Oh, my Lord, I am not eloquent, either in the past or since you have spoken to your servant, but I am slow of speech and of tongue." Then the LORD said to him, "Who has made man's mouth? Who makes him mute, or deaf, or seeing, or blind? Is it not I, the LORD?"

From one perspective we can see how Moses fell into the trap laid in his path by inquiry. Restating to highlight, "God I am not good at speaking. Why did you make me this way, if you want me to lead?" More appropriately direct, Moses did not want to obey God. Though we know not the path desired, Moses wanted to pursue his own course not God's. Moses' questions were an ill-thought-out facade attempting to justify his own wants. However, the lesson is still clear for the present message. God's response almost echoes the words to Job. "Where were you? I make as I see fit." Though God became angry with Moses, God continued to shepherd him towards a spiritual maturity.[29] Asking "why" did not help Moses. God's reassurance of His power comforted not Moses.

---

[29] Exodus 4:14 "Then the anger of the LORD was kindled against Moses and he said, "Is there not Aaron, your brother, the Levite? I know that he can speak well. Behold, he is coming out to meet you, and when he sees you, he will be glad in his heart."

Even when seeking to escape a directive,
answers to "why" provides no solace.

Jumping into the present day and at the risk of
pure repetition, God's answer is not intended as
a universal. God can make you mute, blind,
handless, or however He desires; this passage in
Exodus above, does not state nor imply that God
made you "x" in order for you to do "y". God is
telling Moses; He is aware of Moses' strengths
and limitations and still wants him to lead.
God's communication was comparable to His
words to Job. "I made you and can direct as I
will." God's words to Moses were not, "because I
made you this way"; rather, "I know how you are
made and still want you to do this." God will not
choose you to lead His chosen people.

God is the maker of heaven and earth. God is in
absolute control. God can be considered directly
or indirectly responsible for you. But either
refuge changes not our obligation.   And neither
answer provides grounding for self-elevation.
God did not choose Moses because of inabilities.
God did not cause the inabilities for His glories
to be shown. God chose Moses. Limitations,
inabilities, adversities, illnesses are not signs of
God's glory nor of His will. Your actions and
reactions form a view of glory. Your response
allows others to see God's glory. "What do you
do now?" is the simple restatement.

The normal is not to praise God during or
because of the imperfect human condition. Job,
again provides the guidance.   Job 2:9 "Then his

wife said to him, "Do you still hold fast your integrity? Curse God and die." The desire to live far outstrips the ease at which we will curse God.[30] Even with an acceptance of the human frailty in understanding we would first curse God rather than accept any possible limitation in our comprehension. The unknown becomes more viable than a faith in God's understanding. And in the assignment of supercilious warrior like titles we diminish a belief in the cosmic eternal battle in favor of becoming a General in our own fictious war. Living as I want and desire is not brave.

Moses did not bravely fight against his deficiencies. He did not display courage while struggling to overcome his inabilities. He fought against himself. Moses wanted to obey his own desires not God's. Moses tried to use his conditions to evaluate himself over God.

Again, in the Bible we find the actual battle being clearly defined. It is normal to set your minds on earthly things. It is normal to want to live. It is harmful to elevate the simple into the complex as it changes our focus away from the task. Calling a disease, a deformity, and/or a physical hinderance more than just a part of living is raising the things of earth and demoting

---

[30] It seems likely that the words "Curse God and die." had a cultural meaning which has long been lost. Outside of that explanation I am most comfortable that Job's wife had interspersed pagan believes with God's teaching. She believed that God was awaiting his final surrender before causing his death. Curse God and die, was the only way to appease the spirit that Job had angered.

the things that are above. I believe this is a
universal truth; but for the Christian, Paul's
words to the Colossians are even more stinging.

> Colossians 3:1-2 "If then you have been
> raised with Christ, seek the things that
> are above, where Christ is, seated at the
> right hand of God. Set your minds on
> things that are above, not on things that
> are on earth."

From man's perspective sparrows come and go
but God has not forgotten them.[31] The things
above become harder to focus upon when the
suffering of now is great. But if you have been
raised with Christ this is our new path. Cancer
can do no more than kill the body. Deformities
can do no more than kill the body. Set your
mind on things above and these titles "battles",
"courage", "fights", and "bravery" diminish even
further from relevance. We battle against forces
which do not have our eternal best interest as
their goal.

> Luke 12:4 "I tell you, my friends, do not
> fear those who kill the body, and after that
> have nothing more that they can do."

I do not win against cancer; I do not lose against
cancer. I just live. But, then again, that is all
anyone does … live. Cancer does diminish your
capacity to live, it deprives your body the
opportunity to live. Cancer is like time travel,

---

[31] Luke 12:6 "Are not five sparrows sold for two pennies? And not one
of them is forgotten before God."

only it is just you who is ageing rapidly. As it grows, life does not. If you were to personify cancer, it strangely enough seeks its own death. But it is not a separate thinking, operating being, rather it just is. Just as your heart beats, this mutation just grows. Cancer is a part of you just as much as your hand is.

I can, however, lose my soul.

> Mark 8:34-36 "And calling the crowd to him with his disciples, he said to them, "If anyone would come after me, let him deny himself and take up his cross and follow me. For whoever would save his life will lose it, but whoever loses his life for my sake and the gospel's will save it. For what does it profit a man to gain the whole world and forfeit his soul?"

Part V

Question: Why? Answer: Why not?

The difference between challenging God and a desire to better understand God is often comprised of very thin layers of separation. Understanding your own motives is difficult during normal periods. When you are under stress, it is almost impossible to assess the "why" of yourself. Such as, "Why did I say that?" or "Why did I do that?". Challenging God's choices leads to frustration and probably sin.

Up to this point asking the question "why" has been assigned a damaging negative role when trying to understand God. There is a positive. To over simplify consider these two perspectives. "Why did this happen to me?", will most likely lead to a troublesome path. "Why did God write this in His Bible?", can produce a great deal of personal growth and spiritual maturity.

"Why did God allow this to happen?" Is accurately humanly answered as, "Why not?" While oft presently unsatisfying, this is the Biblical answer. And, "Why did God not tell us much about Jesus' childhood and early adult life?" "Why should He?" is also an acceptable answer but can be misleading. Understanding that there is significance between the questioning of God to gain insight into His ways and commands compared to a challenging "why" upon God, can help point "why" into fruitful territory. The Bible was written to guide, direct, and help us along our task of glorifying our Maker. "These [words] are written so that you may believe."[32] Asking from a position of faith not of challenge, inquiring from a position of humility not of self-righteousness, and desiring to glorify God by obeying His commands[33] are the guideposts for keeping us within the right course.

I am under the impression that we are better off not asking "why" about God's ways. Instead rephrasing questions and inquiries to just simply avoid the word "why" will help guide our thoughts down the correct paths.

For me, the mysteries of the faith[34] are reconcilable; I accept my weakness and in such I become strong.[35] I am comfortable with the answer of "I cannot know." This is not to claim perfection or sinlessness, that reward must wait. Paul's words echo about the world: Romans 7:23 "but I see in my members another law waging

---

[32] John 20:30-31 "Now Jesus did many other signs in the presence of the disciples, which are not written in this book; but these are written so that you may believe that Jesus is the Christ, the Son of God, and that by believing you may have life in his name."
[33] Matthew 28:20 "teaching them to observe all that I have commanded you. And behold, I am with you always, to the end of the age."
[34] 1 Timothy 3:9 "They must hold the mystery of the faith with a clear conscience."
[35] 2 Corinthians 12:10 "For the sake of Christ, then, I am content with weaknesses, insults, hardships, persecutions, and calamities. For when I am weak, then I am strong."

war against the law of my mind and making me captive to the law of sin that dwells in my members." Do not allow the mind to likewise become held captive, reject as you need. It is not in living we battle it is fighting against our own members. It is warfare against yourself that courage must hold. Romans 7:19 "For I do not do the good I want, but the evil I do not want is what I keep on doing." And asking "why" of God can direct the mind where it needs not be. Faith in God's structure and created worlds is not where I stumble and for this, I am grateful.

There is not a battle against yourself but for God's laws. To verbally practice otherwise is an attempt to elevate human experience while usurping God's authority. "For apart from the law, sin lies dead."[36] Courage is not found in living or doing as you desire; it is in the demonstrated of not doing as you want. Heroic actions lay beyond your desires and awaken when the self slumbers. Heroes are made, despite the human condition, as they obey God's commands. Cancer makes not a hero.

Proverbs 8:12-13 "I, wisdom, dwell with prudence, and I find knowledge and discretion. The fear of the LORD is hatred of evil. Pride and arrogance and the way of evil and perverted speech I hate."

---

[36] Romans 7:8 "But sin, seizing an opportunity through the commandment, produced in me all kinds of covetousness. For apart from the law, sin lies dead."

Addendum

Death: A path to comfort.
The edited text from a funeral message of
a young man involved in an accident.

It is with a sad heart and a sorrowful voice I stand here today. For here we are in a place no one desires; but still, we are present. Circumstances, we wish not; pain, we wish were not. Yet here we are. Questions may consume us... confusion might overwhelm. Answers we may lack and still here we are. Moments in time that we wish were not... are recorded. Here we are; together, trying to honor, trying to give and find comfort... moving forward as best we know how. May we find courage to go where we would rather not go but find that we must. We were forced to confront and likewise we are forced to muster strength to continue. Venture where we do not wish... The clock moves but forward... and forward, as you learn again to progress.

This brief message is intended to offer a guide towards comfort; Three reference points, not steps nor a checklist just points of reference.
1) Season of mourning.   2) Questions of doubt, why?   3) The power of pain.

    1) Season of mourning

"We were promised sufferings. They were part of the program. We were even told, 'Blessed are they that mourn,' and I accept it. I've got nothing that I hadn't bargained for. Of course it is different when the thing happens to oneself, not to others, and in reality, not imagination."
— C.S. Lewis, A Grief Observed

Consider this widely used Scripture verse:

> Ecclesiastes 3:1-4 For everything there is a season, and a time for every matter under heaven: a time to be born, and a time to die; a time to plant, and a time to pluck up what is planted; a time to kill, and a time to heal; a time to break down, and a time to build up; a time to weep, and a time to laugh; a time to mourn, and a time to dance;

Feelings can fill the mind; you may find anger, confusion, doubt, frustration, sadness, grief... mourning. There is indeed a time, a season for everything. It is different when the scripture is no longer just read but experienced. Sadly, this is a season of mourning. We no longer wonder as pain and grief is no more imagined.

I turn to the Bible for guidance.

Two Biblical stories come to mind, when living through a season of mourning: The story Lazarus and the story of two brothers Cain and

Able. Perhaps they will seem unconnected at first but they point succinctly to a season.

It is in the story of Lazarus we hear the words, "Jesus wept."[37] Jesus had a good friend named Lazarus who was dying.[38] Lazarus' family had requested Jesus' presence. Before Jesus arrived to the town where Lazarus was, he had died. Now, there is much more to this story but we are told Jesus knew beforehand He was going to heal, raise Lazarus from the dead; yet, Jesus, when he arrived, still wept at the death of Lazarus. There is a season, a time for mourning... even though there was soon to be great joy at this miracle. Jesus wept over the loss of His friend. Christ, Himself, had a season of mourning at the loss of His friend. You should mourn over the loss of a family member, a friend, a human.

Turning to the story of Cain and Able. Cain and Able both brought an offering to God but God did not care for Cain's offering. Again, there is much more to this story but for your season I offer only this highlight. Cain became angry.

> Genesis 4:5-7 "but for Cain and his offering he had no regard. So Cain was very angry, and his face fell. The LORD said to Cain, "Why are you angry, and why has your face fallen? If you do well, will you not be accepted? And if you do not do well, sin is crouching at the door. Its

---

[37] John 11:35 "Jesus wept."
[38] John chapter 11

desire is contrary to you, but you must rule over it."

Crouching is a descriptive word... inferring a trap is set. Your feelings, if allowed to fester, can become a trap of your own making.   Almost all feelings are acceptable, it is how they dwell within you and then if you act upon them even further heartache can be quickly brought about. It is alright to be angry, mad, confused, doubtful.... God told Cain you must rule over your anger, your feelings. To paraphrase, "Cain, your anger will destroy you." In particular, notice that God did not tell Cain not to be angry; He said do not let it (anger) control or guide you. Likewise, you can apply this story to today.

> Ephesians 4:26-27 "Be angry and do not sin; do not let the sun go down on your anger, and give no opportunity to the devil."

This is a season of mourning and suffering. Be angry, be sad, be hurt, be ...   But stay there not. You must rule over it. Bitterness will destroy all where it grows.

The seasons of the year cycle regularly. Gratefully, some seasons of life we may never experience or only experience once. Other people have frequent seasons. Regardless, the mourning is present but the season will need to pass. You must rule over it.

2.) Questions of doubt, Why???

"Why" has led many to stumble into despair and confusion. Too many search for answers when even the best answer could not suffice. Looking again at the Bible for the source of wisdom and understanding. Consider the question: "Why did this happen to me?"

> Matthew 5:45 "so that you may be sons of your Father who is in heaven. For he makes his sun rise on the evil and on the good, and sends rain on the just and on the unjust."

Terrible events happen… world history and personal history graphically describes horrific events. Only a knave would dispute that life is unfair, unjust and even cruel at times. To reference the analogy from Matthew: It rains, when you need it and when you don't. The just and the unjust suffer equally.

The truth revealed here is that, there are unanswerable questions. Again, using the analogy, why did it rain? I don't know. Why… frequently leads into the unanswerable. Why did this occur? Why did this happen to me? One of the hardest truths to accept is, unfortunately, a key to fully living: Things just happen. The rain falls…. The rain falls as it will fall.

We do not like nor want to accept that things just happen or that questions are unanswerable.

But in this simple truth, you can find great comfort. We did not and do not control much about our lives. Who amongst us chose when or where we were born? We did not decide who would be our parents. We didn't decide the century to live. Rather we found ourselves here. Many things have just happened throughout our life and we actually rarely give these items a second thought. Almost everyone has decided at some point to make the best of so much of what we take for granted. Consider if someone challenged the reason they were born Friday the 4th instead of Thursday the 3rd to the point they rejected God? The rain falls and most of the time we accept it as rain falling as it might. Life is really filled with many such decision points of which most we accept. However, it is in the experience of great pain that many people truly begin to ask "why?" In the "small" matters we accept and then the challenge is found in the "great" matters. There is no answer to why it rains on the just and the unjust. Accepting the crushingly painful happenings as unknowable is difficult.

And perhaps now, here in this horrible accident... this will be the greatest moment of such a decision point in your life. Things happen and we must decide our response. The challenge need not be met today nor tomorrow but the challenge will be faced. Allowing the unknowable to be personally accepted... is arduous.

There is nothing to gain by staying planted, rooted in the wanting an answer to an unknowable question, living indefinitely within why ... there is only loss. Rather, here, where you are now... focus instead on, "now what will I do?".

3.) The power of pain

This is an ancient notion, a concept of truth... though difficult to fathom there is power and wisdom to be gained in pain.

Change comes in many ways and manners. Sadly, most significant change is brought on by disaster and pain. This is true both on the political stage as well as in personal lives. Not to be trite, but few can recall what they had for breakfast last week. While the tragic years ago is recalled in great detail even down to a critical few seconds. It is in tragedy that strikes that the greatest change can occur. Tragedy has struck. Rather than why, the question needs to eventually become, "now what?" Will you be consumed by the horror or will move forward? Do you let grief become bitterness or do you let grief power you to betterment? Notice in this next verse how Solomon frames change in the context of wisdom. It is from pain that you can become wise enough to effect significant change.

Solomon was the wisest man and wrote down Godly insights in a book called Ecclesiastes. Perhaps the most famous King found in the Bible is King David. Among his exploits David is known for killing a bear with his hands and a giant, Goliath, with a sling shot. King David's heir to the Israeli kingdom was his son Solomon. One night God asked Solomon what he desired. Solomon asked God for wisdom.[39] Here are some of his words concerning mourning and pain.

> Ecclesiastes 7:2-4 It is better to go to the house of mourning than to go to the house of feasting, for this is the end of all mankind, and the living will lay it to heart. Sorrow is better than laughter, for by sadness of face the heart is made glad. The heart of the wise is in the house of mourning, but the heart of fools is in the house of mirth.

Growth, insight, and yes, wisdom is gained through suffering. Life is comprised of overcoming obstacles…large and small. The guidance gained from merriment is nothing but the heart of a fool. In the house of mourning, you can learn lasting, meaningful insight. Purpose is found in the house of mourning. Mourning lays bare reasons, thoughts, purposes and even goals.

You cannot change the past, only the future is left to change and adjust. It is through mourning that the previously invisible becomes visible…this season of pain can provide you with wisdom. Priorities that were once important may

---

[39] 1st Kings 3:5-13

no longer be, goals that seemed utmost may fade, and even the insignificant may now become important. The heart of the wise is in the house of mourning.

There is an ancient Greek axiom which reflects this same theme,
> "Yea, Zeus, who leadeth men in wisdom's way
> And fixeth fast the law
> That pain is gain."

What do/will you do with the pain? Does it control you? Or, do you control it? Living demands change, small and large. As you have been confronted by death, through no one's desire or fault... Will you change for the better or the worse? According to the Bible, in pain the heart of wisdom is found. In pain and suffering powerful insights can be found. Through the process of pain, you can have a glad heart again.

1.) You are in a season of pain, of mourning. 2.) Within this season, questions of doubt may arise. Comfort can be found in accepting that much is unknowable. 3.) Within your mourning there can be comfort found in wisdom's gain through pain.

May your season of mourning give forth to a time of rebirth and from this into a season of peace. May your pains bring gains which give you lasting comfort.

I'll close these remarks with this verse:

Philippians 4:7-9 And the peace of God, which surpasses all understanding, will guard your hearts and your minds in Christ Jesus. Finally, brothers, whatever is true, whatever is honorable, whatever is just, whatever is pure, whatever is lovely, whatever is commendable, if there is any excellence, if there is anything worthy of praise, think about these things. What you have learned and received and heard and seen in me—practice these things, and the God of peace will be with you.

www.ingramcontent.com/pod-product-compliance
Lightning Source LLC
Chambersburg PA
CBHW072340270726
48659CB00022B/2081